This
Blood Pressure
Log Book
Belongs To:

_____

_____

_____

© 2019 Inigo Creations

DATE	TIME	SYSTOLIC (UPPER #)	DIASTOLIC (LOWER #)	HEART RATE (PULSE)	NOTES

DATE	TIME	SYSTOLIC (UPPER #)	DIASTOLIC (LOWER #)	HEART RATE (PULSE)	NOTES

DATE	TIME	SYSTOLIC (UPPER #)	DIASTOLIC (LOWER #)	HEART RATE (PULSE)	NOTES

DATE	TIME	SYSTOLIC (UPPER #)	DIASTOLIC (LOWER #)	HEART RATE (PULSE)	NOTES

DATE	TIME	SYSTOLIC (UPPER #)	DIASTOLIC (LOWER #)	HEART RATE (PULSE)	NOTES

DATE	TIME	SYSTOLIC (UPPER #)	DIASTOLIC (LOWER #)	HEART RATE (PULSE)	NOTES

DATE	TIME	SYSTOLIC (UPPER #)	DIASTOLIC (LOWER #)	HEART RATE (PULSE)	NOTES

DATE	TIME	SYSTOLIC (UPPER #)	DIASTOLIC (LOWER #)	HEART RATE (PULSE)	NOTES

DATE	TIME	SYSTOLIC (UPPER #)	DIASTOLIC (LOWER #)	HEART RATE (PULSE)	NOTES

DATE	TIME	SYSTOLIC (UPPER #)	DIASTOLIC (LOWER #)	HEART RATE (PULSE)	NOTES

DATE	TIME	SYSTOLIC (UPPER #)	DIASTOLIC (LOWER #)	HEART RATE (PULSE)	NOTES

DATE	TIME	SYSTOLIC (UPPER #)	DIASTOLIC (LOWER #)	HEART RATE (PULSE)	NOTES

DATE	TIME	SYSTOLIC (UPPER #)	DIASTOLIC (LOWER #)	HEART RATE (PULSE)	NOTES

DATE	TIME	SYSTOLIC (UPPER #)	DIASTOLIC (LOWER #)	HEART RATE (PULSE)	NOTES

DATE	TIME	SYSTOLIC (UPPER #)	DIASTOLIC (LOWER #)	HEART RATE (PULSE)	NOTES

DATE	TIME	SYSTOLIC (UPPER #)	DIASTOLIC (LOWER #)	HEART RATE (PULSE)	NOTES

DATE	TIME	SYSTOLIC (UPPER #)	DIASTOLIC (LOWER #)	HEART RATE (PULSE)	NOTES

DATE	TIME	SYSTOLIC (UPPER #)	DIASTOLIC (LOWER #)	HEART RATE (PULSE)	NOTES

DATE	TIME	SYSTOLIC (UPPER #)	DIASTOLIC (LOWER #)	HEART RATE (PULSE)	NOTES

DATE	TIME	SYSTOLIC (UPPER #)	DIASTOLIC (LOWER #)	HEART RATE (PULSE)	NOTES

DATE	TIME	SYSTOLIC (UPPER #)	DIASTOLIC (LOWER #)	HEART RATE (PULSE)	NOTES

DATE	TIME	SYSTOLIC (UPPER #)	DIASTOLIC (LOWER #)	HEART RATE (PULSE)	NOTES

DATE	TIME	SYSTOLIC (UPPER #)	DIASTOLIC (LOWER #)	HEART RATE (PULSE)	NOTES

DATE	TIME	SYSTOLIC (UPPER #)	DIASTOLIC (LOWER #)	HEART RATE (PULSE)	NOTES

DATE	TIME	SYSTOLIC (UPPER #)	DIASTOLIC (LOWER #)	HEART RATE (PULSE)	NOTES

DATE	TIME	SYSTOLIC (UPPER #)	DIASTOLIC (LOWER #)	HEART RATE (PULSE)	NOTES

DATE	TIME	SYSTOLIC (UPPER #)	DIASTOLIC (LOWER #)	HEART RATE (PULSE)	NOTES

DATE	TIME	SYSTOLIC (UPPER #)	DIASTOLIC (LOWER #)	HEART RATE (PULSE)	NOTES

DATE	TIME	SYSTOLIC (UPPER #)	DIASTOLIC (LOWER #)	HEART RATE (PULSE)	NOTES

DATE	TIME	SYSTOLIC (UPPER #)	DIASTOLIC (LOWER #)	HEART RATE (PULSE)	NOTES

DATE	TIME	SYSTOLIC (UPPER #)	DIASTOLIC (LOWER #)	HEART RATE (PULSE)	NOTES

DATE	TIME	SYSTOLIC (UPPER #)	DIASTOLIC (LOWER #)	HEART RATE (PULSE)	NOTES

DATE	TIME	SYSTOLIC (UPPER #)	DIASTOLIC (LOWER #)	HEART RATE (PULSE)	NOTES

DATE	TIME	SYSTOLIC (UPPER #)	DIASTOLIC (LOWER #)	HEART RATE (PULSE)	NOTES

DATE	TIME	SYSTOLIC (UPPER #)	DIASTOLIC (LOWER #)	HEART RATE (PULSE)	NOTES

DATE	TIME	SYSTOLIC (UPPER #)	DIASTOLIC (LOWER #)	HEART RATE (PULSE)	NOTES

DATE	TIME	SYSTOLIC (UPPER #)	DIASTOLIC (LOWER #)	HEART RATE (PULSE)	NOTES

DATE	TIME	SYSTOLIC (UPPER #)	DIASTOLIC (LOWER #)	HEART RATE (PULSE)	NOTES

DATE	TIME	SYSTOLIC (UPPER #)	DIASTOLIC (LOWER #)	HEART RATE (PULSE)	NOTES

DATE	TIME	SYSTOLIC (UPPER #)	DIASTOLIC (LOWER #)	HEART RATE (PULSE)	NOTES

DATE	TIME	SYSTOLIC (UPPER #)	DIASTOLIC (LOWER #)	HEART RATE (PULSE)	NOTES

DATE	TIME	SYSTOLIC (UPPER #)	DIASTOLIC (LOWER #)	HEART RATE (PULSE)	NOTES

DATE	TIME	SYSTOLIC (UPPER #)	DIASTOLIC (LOWER #)	HEART RATE (PULSE)	NOTES

DATE	TIME	SYSTOLIC (UPPER #)	DIASTOLIC (LOWER #)	HEART RATE (PULSE)	NOTES

DATE	TIME	SYSTOLIC (UPPER #)	DIASTOLIC (LOWER #)	HEART RATE (PULSE)	NOTES

DATE	TIME	SYSTOLIC (UPPER #)	DIASTOLIC (LOWER #)	HEART RATE (PULSE)	NOTES

DATE	TIME	SYSTOLIC (UPPER #)	DIASTOLIC (LOWER #)	HEART RATE (PULSE)	NOTES

DATE	TIME	SYSTOLIC (UPPER #)	DIASTOLIC (LOWER #)	HEART RATE (PULSE)	NOTES

DATE	TIME	SYSTOLIC (UPPER #)	DIASTOLIC (LOWER #)	HEART RATE (PULSE)	NOTES

DATE	TIME	SYSTOLIC (UPPER #)	DIASTOLIC (LOWER #)	HEART RATE (PULSE)	NOTES

DATE	TIME	SYSTOLIC (UPPER #)	DIASTOLIC (LOWER #)	HEART RATE (PULSE)	NOTES

DATE	TIME	SYSTOLIC (UPPER #)	DIASTOLIC (LOWER #)	HEART RATE (PULSE)	NOTES

DATE	TIME	SYSTOLIC (UPPER #)	DIASTOLIC (LOWER #)	HEART RATE (PULSE)	NOTES

DATE	TIME	SYSTOLIC (UPPER #)	DIASTOLIC (LOWER #)	HEART RATE (PULSE)	NOTES

DATE	TIME	SYSTOLIC (UPPER #)	DIASTOLIC (LOWER #)	HEART RATE (PULSE)	NOTES

DATE	TIME	SYSTOLIC (UPPER #)	DIASTOLIC (LOWER #)	HEART RATE (PULSE)	NOTES

DATE	TIME	SYSTOLIC (UPPER #)	DIASTOLIC (LOWER #)	HEART RATE (PULSE)	NOTES

DATE	TIME	SYSTOLIC (UPPER #)	DIASTOLIC (LOWER #)	HEART RATE (PULSE)	NOTES

DATE	TIME	SYSTOLIC (UPPER #)	DIASTOLIC (LOWER #)	HEART RATE (PULSE)	NOTES

DATE	TIME	SYSTOLIC (UPPER #)	DIASTOLIC (LOWER #)	HEART RATE (PULSE)	NOTES

DATE	TIME	SYSTOLIC (UPPER #)	DIASTOLIC (LOWER #)	HEART RATE (PULSE)	NOTES

DATE	TIME	SYSTOLIC (UPPER #)	DIASTOLIC (LOWER #)	HEART RATE (PULSE)	NOTES

DATE	TIME	SYSTOLIC (UPPER #)	DIASTOLIC (LOWER #)	HEART RATE (PULSE)	NOTES

DATE	TIME	SYSTOLIC (UPPER #)	DIASTOLIC (LOWER #)	HEART RATE (PULSE)	NOTES

DATE	TIME	SYSTOLIC (UPPER #)	DIASTOLIC (LOWER #)	HEART RATE (PULSE)	NOTES

DATE	TIME	SYSTOLIC (UPPER #)	DIASTOLIC (LOWER #)	HEART RATE (PULSE)	NOTES

DATE	TIME	SYSTOLIC (UPPER #)	DIASTOLIC (LOWER #)	HEART RATE (PULSE)	NOTES

DATE	TIME	SYSTOLIC (UPPER #)	DIASTOLIC (LOWER #)	HEART RATE (PULSE)	NOTES

DATE	TIME	SYSTOLIC (UPPER #)	DIASTOLIC (LOWER #)	HEART RATE (PULSE)	NOTES

DATE	TIME	SYSTOLIC (UPPER #)	DIASTOLIC (LOWER #)	HEART RATE (PULSE)	NOTES

DATE	TIME	SYSTOLIC (UPPER #)	DIASTOLIC (LOWER #)	HEART RATE (PULSE)	NOTES

DATE	TIME	SYSTOLIC (UPPER #)	DIASTOLIC (LOWER #)	HEART RATE (PULSE)	NOTES

DATE	TIME	SYSTOLIC (UPPER #)	DIASTOLIC (LOWER #)	HEART RATE (PULSE)	NOTES

DATE	TIME	SYSTOLIC (UPPER #)	DIASTOLIC (LOWER #)	HEART RATE (PULSE)	NOTES

DATE	TIME	SYSTOLIC (UPPER #)	DIASTOLIC (LOWER #)	HEART RATE (PULSE)	NOTES

DATE	TIME	SYSTOLIC (UPPER #)	DIASTOLIC (LOWER #)	HEART RATE (PULSE)	NOTES

DATE	TIME	SYSTOLIC (UPPER #)	DIASTOLIC (LOWER #)	HEART RATE (PULSE)	NOTES

DATE	TIME	SYSTOLIC (UPPER #)	DIASTOLIC (LOWER #)	HEART RATE (PULSE)	NOTES

DATE	TIME	SYSTOLIC (UPPER #)	DIASTOLIC (LOWER #)	HEART RATE (PULSE)	NOTES

DATE	TIME	SYSTOLIC (UPPER #)	DIASTOLIC (LOWER #)	HEART RATE (PULSE)	NOTES

DATE	TIME	SYSTOLIC (UPPER #)	DIASTOLIC (LOWER #)	HEART RATE (PULSE)	NOTES

DATE	TIME	SYSTOLIC (UPPER #)	DIASTOLIC (LOWER #)	HEART RATE (PULSE)	NOTES

DATE	TIME	SYSTOLIC (UPPER #)	DIASTOLIC (LOWER #)	HEART RATE (PULSE)	NOTES

DATE	TIME	SYSTOLIC (UPPER #)	DIASTOLIC (LOWER #)	HEART RATE (PULSE)	NOTES

DATE	TIME	SYSTOLIC (UPPER #)	DIASTOLIC (LOWER #)	HEART RATE (PULSE)	NOTES

DATE	TIME	SYSTOLIC (UPPER #)	DIASTOLIC (LOWER #)	HEART RATE (PULSE)	NOTES

DATE	TIME	SYSTOLIC (UPPER #)	DIASTOLIC (LOWER #)	HEART RATE (PULSE)	NOTES

DATE	TIME	SYSTOLIC (UPPER #)	DIASTOLIC (LOWER #)	HEART RATE (PULSE)	NOTES

DATE	TIME	SYSTOLIC (UPPER #)	DIASTOLIC (LOWER #)	HEART RATE (PULSE)	NOTES

DATE	TIME	SYSTOLIC (UPPER #)	DIASTOLIC (LOWER #)	HEART RATE (PULSE)	NOTES

DATE	TIME	SYSTOLIC (UPPER #)	DIASTOLIC (LOWER #)	HEART RATE (PULSE)	NOTES

DATE	TIME	SYSTOLIC (UPPER #)	DIASTOLIC (LOWER #)	HEART RATE (PULSE)	NOTES

DATE	TIME	SYSTOLIC (UPPER #)	DIASTOLIC (LOWER #)	HEART RATE (PULSE)	NOTES

DATE	TIME	SYSTOLIC (UPPER #)	DIASTOLIC (LOWER #)	HEART RATE (PULSE)	NOTES

DATE	TIME	SYSTOLIC (UPPER #)	DIASTOLIC (LOWER #)	HEART RATE (PULSE)	NOTES

DATE	TIME	SYSTOLIC (UPPER #)	DIASTOLIC (LOWER #)	HEART RATE (PULSE)	NOTES

DATE	TIME	SYSTOLIC (UPPER #)	DIASTOLIC (LOWER #)	HEART RATE (PULSE)	NOTES

DATE	TIME	SYSTOLIC (UPPER #)	DIASTOLIC (LOWER #)	HEART RATE (PULSE)	NOTES

DATE	TIME	SYSTOLIC (UPPER #)	DIASTOLIC (LOWER #)	HEART RATE (PULSE)	NOTES

DATE	TIME	SYSTOLIC (UPPER #)	DIASTOLIC (LOWER #)	HEART RATE (PULSE)	NOTES

Notes

Notes

Notes

Notes

Notes

Notes

Notes

Made in the USA
Monee, IL
06 March 2023

29312984R00066